OVERVIEW

OF THE

HIV/AIDS

EPIDEMIC

DR KENNETH WOOD

This book was dedicated to
you.

I believe you will know how to
prevent HIV/AIDS after reading
this book

CONTENTS TABLE

INTRODUCTION

HIV/AIDS is a pandemic that has altered the course of human history. Knowing the virus's history and origins is necessary to comprehend the virus and its effects. HIV/AIDS has devastated communities all over the world since the early 1980s. It is still a significant public health issue today, especially in low-income areas. Unfortunately, many people continue to lack access to testing, treatment, and education.

The virus still disproportionately affects vulnerable populations in spite of our best efforts. Stigma and discrimination exacerbate the problem, frequently preventing access to care. Without a doubt, a lot has changed since those early days, but work remains. We'll go into more detail about the symptoms, transmission, and treatment of HIV/AIDS in the sections that follow.

CAUSES OF HIV/AIDS

The Human Immunodeficiency Virus (HIV) itself is the main contributor to HIV/AIDS. Blood, semen, vaginal fluids, and breast milk are the bodily fluids most commonly used in the transmission of HIV. Unprotected sexual contact, sharing contaminated needles or syringes, and mother-to-child transmission during childbirth or breastfeeding are common methods of transmission.

It's crucial to remember that casual contact, such as hugging, shaking hands, or using the same toilet, cannot spread HIV. Insect bites, water, or the air do not spread the virus.

Additional elements that aid in the spread of HIV/AIDS include:

1. Unprotected sex: Having sex without the use of condoms or other barrier techniques can raise the risk of HIV transmission.

2. Sharing contaminated needles, syringes, or other drug paraphernalia is a

common way for HIV to spread among injection drug users.

3. Mother-to-child transmission: If precautions are not taken, HIV-positive pregnant women may infect their unborn children during delivery or through breastfeeding.

4. Limited access to healthcare can impede early diagnosis and effective management of the infection. This includes limited access to HIV testing, treatment, and education.

5. Stigma and discrimination: Individuals may be reluctant to seek testing, care,

and support out of a fear of judgment or discrimination based on their HIV status, which can contribute to the virus's spread.

In order to stop further transmission of the virus and enhance general health outcomes, it is essential to promote safe sexual behavior, make HIV testing and treatment accessible, and support those who already have the virus.

TRANSMISSION AND PREVENTION

It is incredible how HIV, a virus discovered only 40 years ago, has sparked a worldwide epidemic that has killed millions of people. AIDS, a condition in which the body is unable to fight off infections and diseases, can result from HIV's attack on the immune system. Blood, semen, vaginal fluids, and breast milk are among the bodily fluids most commonly used in the transmission of HIV.

Safe sexual behavior, the use of condoms, adherence to general precautionary measures, and refraining from sharing needles when injecting drugs are all preventative measures that can be taken to lessen the spread of the virus. Although the number of new HIV infections has decreased as a result of these actions, prevention challenges still exist. A few of the many factors that make prevention challenging are lack of access to quality healthcare, education, and poverty.

Preventing, managing, and treating HIV is a serious issue that requires our full attention. We can contribute to eradicating the stigma associated with the disease by treating people living with HIV with respect and dignity. It is crucial to keep fighting for the rights of those affected by HIV/AIDS and to make resources more accessible to all those who need them. We can improve the world for everyone if we work together.

SYMPTOMS AND DIAGNOSIS

Knowing the warning signs and symptoms of acute HIV infection is crucial because an early diagnosis can improve prognosis. Acute HIV infection symptoms can resemble flu-like symptoms. Fever, exhaustion, aches in the muscles, and sore throat are possible symptoms. Swollen lymph nodes, rash, and mouth ulcers are a few additional symptoms that could occur. Within two to four weeks of HIV exposure, these symptoms may start to show up and may continue for a few weeks.

However, not everyone will show signs of an acute HIV infection. There may go years without any symptoms in some circumstances. During this time, the virus will keep weakening the immune system and advancing HIV. HIV Development Persistent fever, exhaustion, night sweats, diarrhea, and weight loss are a few symptoms that may be present. HIV can develop into AIDS, a serious illness in which the immune system is severely harmed, if it is not treated.

Early diagnosis is therefore essential. A confidential and anonymous HIV test is available. Regulatory authorities-approved test kits are also available for use in at-home testing. Early diagnosis allows for the quick start of antiretroviral therapy (ART), which entails daily medication to suppress the virus.

In conclusion, identifying the symptoms and signs of acute HIV infection is crucial for ensuring a timely diagnosis. Early diagnosis improves prognosis and increases ART effectiveness. Therefore, it is imperative to have regular tests, especially if engaging in risky behavior. Keep in mind that getting tested benefits you personally as well as your partner and the community.

TREATMENT AND MANAGEMENT

Antiretroviral therapy (ART) is the treatment of choice for managing HIV/AIDS. People with HIV are able to live long and healthy lives thanks to ART. But there's a catch: you have to take the medication consistently, without fail, each and every day.

People who lead busy lives or who are unable to afford their medication may find this challenging. Many people who begin taking ART might also experience side effects, which can include everything from nausea to headaches. ART is still the best tool we have for controlling the virus despite these difficulties.

But just because we have the resources to control HIV/AIDS doesn't mean everyone has access to them equally. People who are poor or marginalized may find it difficult to get the medical care and medications they require to stay healthy. Additionally, HIV-positive people continue to face significant stigma and discrimination in some communities. People may find it difficult to get the care they require as a result, or to go about their daily lives without worrying about being judged.

But there is some good news on the way. In an effort to control HIV/AIDS and eventually find a cure, researchers are constantly creating new medications and management techniques. Additionally, a large number of activists and supporters are working to ensure that people with HIV/AIDS have access to care and treatment as well as a life free from prejudice and marginalization.

EFFECTS OF HIV/AIDS

Worldwide, HIV/AIDS has had a terrible effect on people, families, and communities. The effects of this epidemic are wide-ranging and go beyond health. Living with HIV/AIDS has significant and lasting social, economic, and psychological ramifications.

The toll HIV/AIDS takes on people and their families is among its most significant effects. The disease's physical symptoms can be severely disabling, which lowers a person's quality of life in general. Families are frequently financially burdened and vulnerable as a result of the loss of productivity brought on by illness and the subsequent medical expenses. In addition, the emotional strain of seeing a loved one struggle with this illness can be crippling, resulting in severe distress and anxiety.

Additionally, communities are hardest hit by the HIV/AIDS epidemic. Affected people become more stigmatized as a result of the disease's outbreak, which disturbs the social order. Social exclusion and isolation caused by discrimination and prejudice against people living with HIV/AIDS exacerbate the problems faced by the affected communities. Additionally, the loss of productive citizens brought on by the early deaths brought on by HIV/AIDS impedes the growth and stability of the economy.

The effects of HIV/AIDS go beyond what they have on people and communities right away. Significant economic ramifications result from it, especially in low- and middle-income nations. The cost of offering medical care, preventative services, and antiretroviral therapy places a significant strain on already overburdened healthcare systems. Additionally, the epidemic's loss of potential earnings and human capital prevents economic development and feeds the cycle of poverty.

The global health crisis of HIV/AIDS has significant social repercussions. Beyond its effects on health, HIV/AIDS raises a number of social issues that continue to pose difficulties for people in communities and societies around the world. Here are some major social problems linked to HIV/AIDS:

1. Stigma and Discrimination: One of the biggest social problems with HIV/AIDS is the ongoing stigma and prejudice that those who have the virus must deal with. People living with HIV/AIDS frequently experience prejudice, exclusion, and even violence as a result of misunderstandings and fears about

the illness, which feeds feelings of isolation and shame.

2. Healthcare Access: The inequitable access to healthcare services for those living with HIV/AIDS is a second social issue. Accessibility is often hampered by poor healthcare infrastructure, expensive treatments, and resource shortages, which disproportionately affect marginalized communities. This contributes to the virus' continued spread and exacerbates already-present social injustices.

3. Education and Awareness: For the eradication of preconceptions and the reduction of discriminatory behavior,

it is essential to raise awareness and provide accurate information about HIV/AIDS. Lack of accurate information about HIV transmission and prevention creates social problems by allowing stigmatizing beliefs to persist. In order to address this issue, comprehensive sex education in schools and community outreach programs are crucial.

4. Gender Inequality: In environments with scarce resources, HIV/AIDS disproportionately affects women and girls. Inequality between the sexes, which includes unequal power dynamics, restricted educational opportunities, and economic dependence, has a big impact on how

susceptible people are to infection. Fighting the social effects of HIV/AIDS requires addressing gender disparities and empowering women and girls.

5. Community Support and Resources: Communities are essential in providing HIV/AIDS patients with support networks. Social problems develop when these support systems are absent or inaccessible, depriving those who need them of the necessary emotional, monetary, and medical resources. For reducing social isolation and improving general wellbeing, it is essential to strengthen community-based organizations and support inclusive environments.

Governments, healthcare providers, civil society organizations, and communities must work together to address these social issues in a multifaceted manner. Effectively combating the social effects of HIV/AIDS depends on promoting advocacy, defending human rights, and fostering inclusive societies. We can combat stigma, discrimination, and inequality related to HIV/AIDS by banding together and making sure that everyone has access to the care and support they require to live healthy and fulfilling lives.

CONCLUSION

Human Immunodeficiency Virus/Acquired Immunodeficiency Syndrome, also known as HIV/AIDS, is a global health issue that has impacted millions of people across the globe. HIV is a virus that attacks the immune system of the body, specifically targeting CD4 cells, which are essential for defending the body against illnesses and infections. If left untreated, HIV can develop into AIDS over time, which is characterized by a severely weakened immune system that leaves sufferers more susceptible to opportunistic infections and specific cancers.

HIV primarily spreads through sexual contact, sharing needles or other drug paraphernalia, mother-to-child transmission during childbirth or breastfeeding, and blood transfusions with infected blood (though this is uncommon in most developed countries due to stringent blood screening). It's important to remember that casual contact, such as hugs, handshakes, or sharing of household items, cannot spread HIV.

Beyond its physical consequences, HIV/AIDS has a significant negative social, economic, and psychological impact. HIV/AIDS patients frequently experience stigma, prejudice, and restricted access to medical care and support services. Additionally, marginalized groups like women, young people, and residents of low-income communities bear an outsized share of the disease's burden.

The prognosis for people living with HIV/AIDS has significantly improved as a result of recent advances in medical treatment. By successfully suppressing the virus and enabling patients to live long, healthy lives, antiretroviral therapy (ART) has revolutionized the management of this condition. In order to stop new infections, prevention strategies are essential, such as using clean needles, engaging in safe sex, and choosing HIV testing and counseling.

The fight against HIV/AIDS includes extensive education and awareness campaigns, promoting access to cost-effective, high-quality healthcare, standing up for the rights of people living with the disease, and working to lessen the stigma attached to it. To address this ongoing global health crisis, governments, international organizations, and civil society must work together and engage in global initiatives, research, and collaborations.

In conclusion, HIV/AIDS remains a major problem, but we can work toward a world in which it doesn't endanger public health by investing in more research, prevention programs, and treatment access.